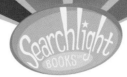

Searchlight BOOKS™

Celebrating Failure

Great

Medicine Fails

Barbara Krasner

Lerner Publications ◆ Minneapolis

Lerner Publications Company
An imprint of Lerner Publishing Group, Inc.
241 First Avenue North
Minneapolis, MN 55401 USA

For reading levels and more information, look up this title at www.lernerbooks.com.

Main body text set in Adrianna Regular.
Typeface provided by Chank.

Library of Congress Cataloging-in-Publication Data

Names: Krasner, Barbara, author.
Title: Great medicine fails / Barbara Krasner.
Description: Minneapolis : Lerner Publications, [2020] | Series: Searchlight books. Celebrating failure | Audience: Ages 8–12. | Audience: Grades 4 to 6. | Includes bibliographical references and index.
Identifiers: LCCN 2019005182 | ISBN 9781541577350 (lb : alk. paper)
Subjects: LCSH: Medical errors—History—Juvenile literature. | Medicine—History—Juvenile literature.
Classification: LCC R729.8 .K73275 2020 | DDC 610.9—dc23

LC record available at https://lccn.loc.gov/2019005182

Manufactured in the United States of America
1-46757-47748-5/29/2019

Contents

Chapter 1

A BAD NIGHT FOR GEORGE WASHINGTON

December 12, 1799, was a cold, wet day in Virginia. Retired US president George Washington still wanted to check up on trees, animals, and workers on his large farm, Mount Vernon. He spent five hours on horseback in the snow and rain. He remained in his wet clothes during dinner.

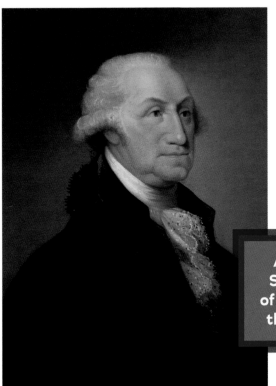

American painter Edward Savage made this portrait of George Washington about three years before he died.

WASHINGTON FELL ILL AT MOUNT VERNON, HIS HOME IN VIRGINIA, IN LATE 1799.

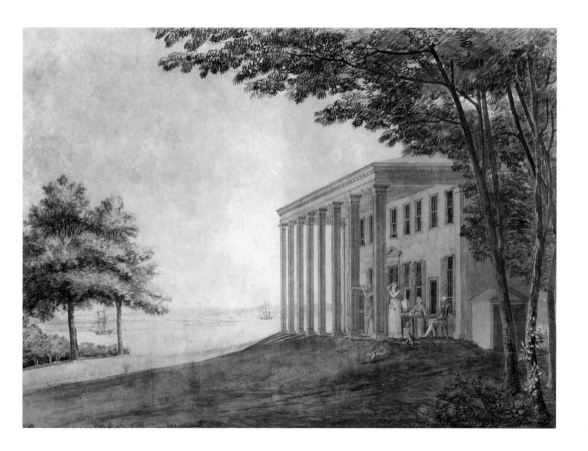

The next morning, Washington had a sore throat. But he again spent another snowy day outdoors. That night, he awoke at three in the morning. He told his wife, Martha, that he was ill. He had trouble breathing and talking.

He asked George Rawlins, Mount Vernon's manager, to bleed him. Bleeding, or bloodletting, had been a common medical practice since ancient times. Doctors believed that getting rid of "bad" blood would create balance in the body and heal the patient. Even though the overseer was not a trained doctor, Washington offered him his arm. The overseer cut a vein to allow some blood to flow out.

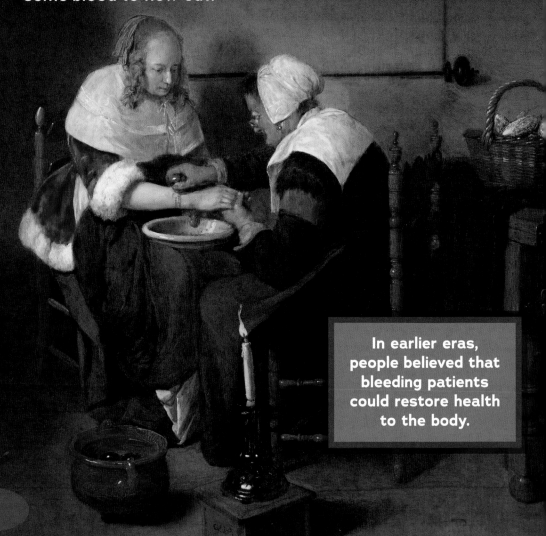

In earlier eras, people believed that bleeding patients could restore health to the body.

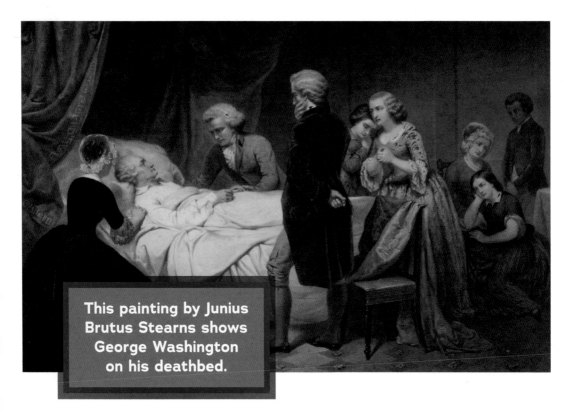

This painting by Junius Brutus Stearns shows George Washington on his deathbed.

Washington's doctor came at nine o'clock. He called in two other doctors to help. They bled Washington repeatedly. They tried other remedies to bring Washington back to health. They had him gargle with molasses mixed with vinegar and butter. They had him inhale the steam of hot water mixed with vinegar. They swabbed his throat with a powder made of crushed emerald-green beetles. None of these remedies worked.

George Washington died at 10:20 p.m. on December 14. By then, because of the bleeding, he had lost 40 percent of his blood.

An Imperfect Practice

No one is sure what made George Washington sick in the first place. Some modern doctors think a virus might have infected his tongue. Modern doctors also think that by draining 40 percent of Washington's blood, his doctors made him even sicker.

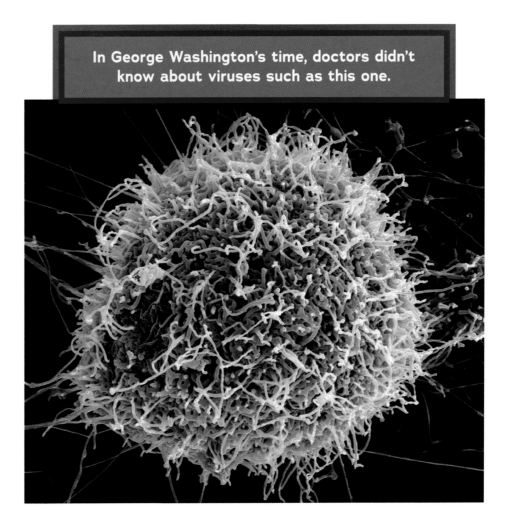

In George Washington's time, doctors didn't know about viruses such as this one.

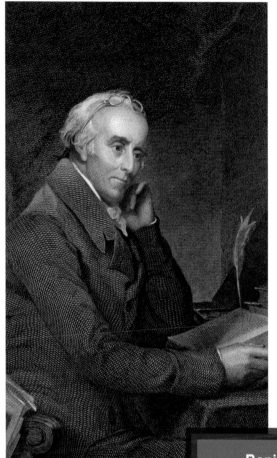

Doctors in Washington's time had limited medical knowledge. They did not know about viruses and bacteria. They did not have medicines such as antibiotics. They often used treatments that were harmful, such as bleeding.

Benjamin Rush was a physician and early leader of the United States. Like George Washington's doctors, he often bled his patients.

DESPITE HIGH-LEVEL TRAINING AND HIGH-TECH EQUIPMENT, DOCTORS SOMETIMES MAKE MISTAKES.

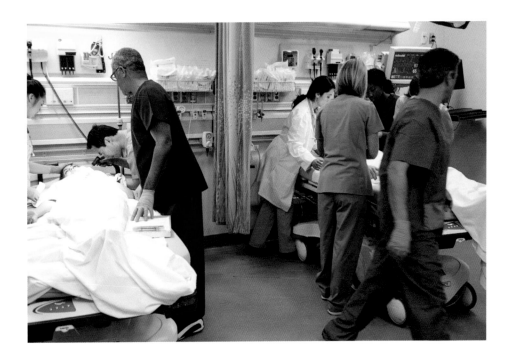

Doctors still make mistakes and bad decisions. Medical mistakes can be deadly, but sometimes they lead to advances in medicine. Sometimes mistakes lead to new discoveries. Sometimes they change training for doctors, nurses, and other medical staff. Mistakes might also lead to new rules that improve patient care.

The Road to Failure

Ignaz Semmelweis (*below left*) was an obstetrician, a doctor who cares for pregnant mothers and their babies. In the 1840s, he worked at a hospital in Vienna, Austria. Many newborns there died from puerperal fever. But Semmelweis found that when health workers washed their hands before delivering babies, rates of puerperal fever dropped greatly.

Semmelweis advised other doctors to wash their hands before treating patients. Most of them ignored him. His advice offended some of them. They thought he was calling them dirty and blaming them for killing patients. Semmelweis failed to convince doctors that handwashing saved lives.

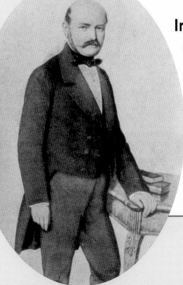

In the late nineteenth century, other doctors learned that bacteria could cause disease. They figured out that handwashing prevents the spread of disease-causing bacteria. Semmelweis had been right all along. But no one recognized his contribution to medicine until long after his death.

Chapter 2

OOPS! ACCIDENTAL DISCOVERIES

In 1895, German physicist Wilhelm Roentgen was studying vacuum tubes. He covered a glass tube with black paper and jolted it with electric current. A strange green light glowed on a nearby screen. Roentgen realized that rays of energy had passed through the black paper onto the screen. He called them X-rays.

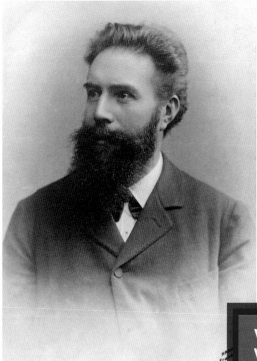

While studying vacuum tubes, William Roentgen accidentally discovered X-rays.

By experimenting, he found that X-rays could pass through certain objects and not others. In one experiment, Roentgen had his wife put her hand on photographic film. Roentgen exposed her hand to X-rays. The rays passed through her skin and muscles but not through the bones in her hand or her wedding ring. A picture of the bones and ring appeared on the film.

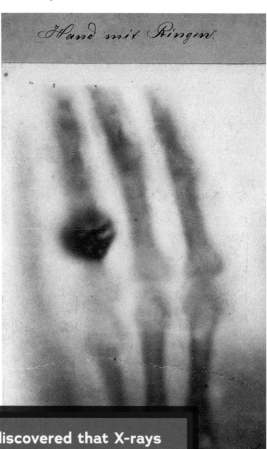

Roentgen discovered that X-rays could pass through skin and muscle to show bones inside the body.

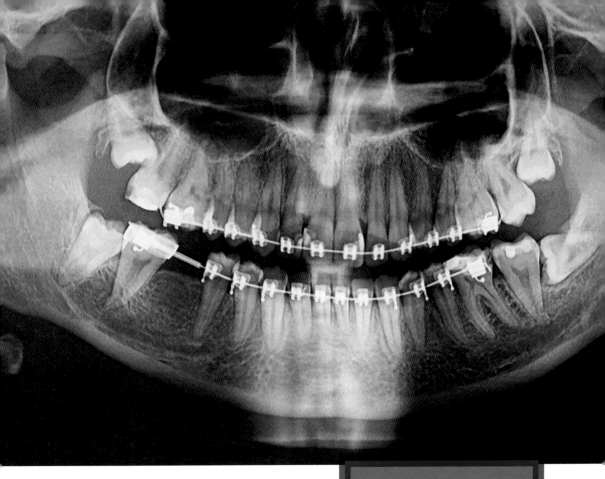

Dentists use X-rays to see how teeth line up inside the upper and lower jaw.

Roentgen was not a doctor. He had not been looking for a medical breakthrough. But doctors quickly realized the importance of his discovery. X-rays allowed them to see inside the human body without performing surgery. They used X-rays to find broken bones, tumors, cavities in teeth, and other medical problems.

The Wrong Transistor

Wilson Greatbatch taught electrical engineering at the University of Buffalo in New York. In 1956, he wanted to

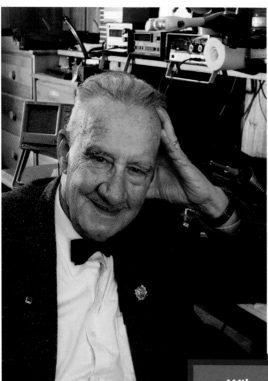

build a machine that would record electrical signals in the human heart. By mistake, he attached the wrong transistor to his invention. This transistor made the machine produce steady bursts of electricity instead of record them. The electrical signals matched the beat of the human heart.

Wilson Greatbatch's mistake led to the creation of the pacemaker, a lifesaving device.

By accident, Greatbatch had invented a pacemaker. This machine corrects an irregular heartbeat. Doctors had used pacemakers before, but they were big and bulky. Patients strapped them to their bodies. Greatbatch's device was just a few centimeters wide. It was small enough to fit inside a patient's chest. In 1960, doctors implanted the first pacemaker into a human patient. Since then, Greatbatch's mistake has saved millions of lives.

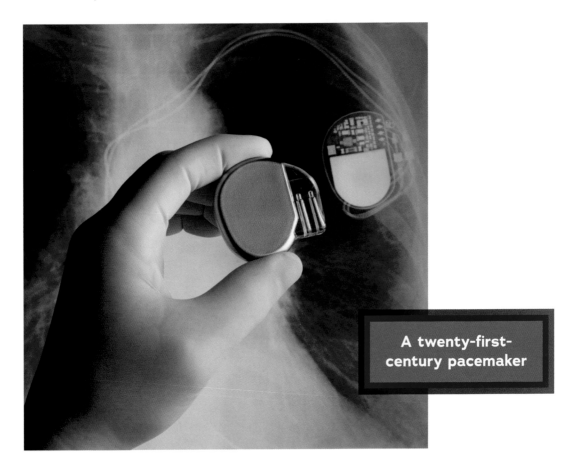

A twenty-first-century pacemaker

Failing Upward

In 1928, Scottish scientist Alexander Fleming (*below left*) discovered a mold called penicillin. He wanted to turn it into an antibiotic. But his experiments kept failing. When he tried to turn penicillin into medicine, the mold lost its power. Frustrated, Fleming stopped experimenting.

In 1938, British researchers Howard Florey and Ernst Chain learned about Fleming's experiments. They figured out how to turn penicillin into medicine.

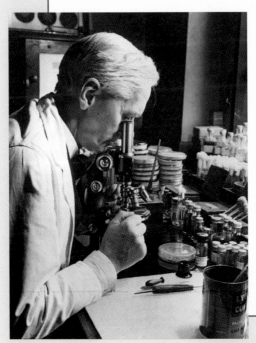

During World War II (1939–1945), doctors gave penicillin to wounded soldiers. It killed the bacteria that had infected their wounds.

Penicillin also kills bacteria that causes pneumonia, meningitis, and other diseases. It is a lifesaving drug.

Chapter 3

TRAGEDY BRINGS BETTER CARE

In February 1976, a small plane crashed in a cornfield in Nebraska. The pilot was James Styner, a surgeon. He and his family were returning home to Nebraska from California. The crash killed Styner's wife. He and his four children were badly injured.

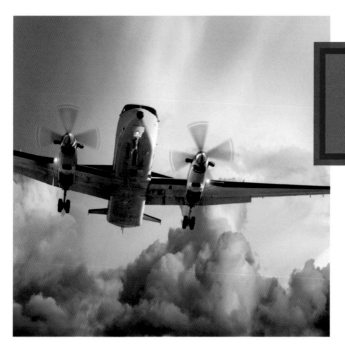

A tragic airplane crash led to the creation of a lifesaving system.

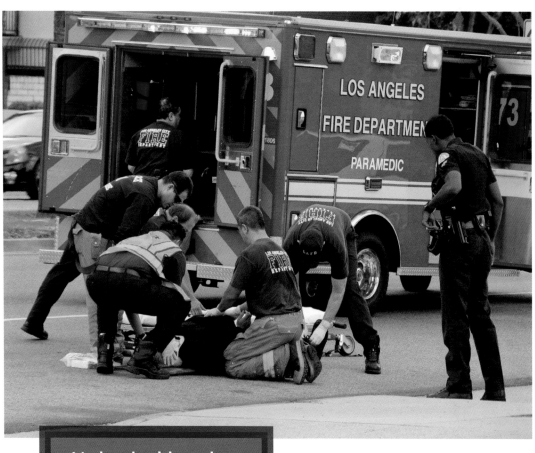

Styner flagged down a passing driver. He took the five survivors to a local hospital. But the small hospital was not equipped to handle such a serious emergency. Styner was angry. He thought that US hospitals and medical clinics needed a system for treating severely injured patients.

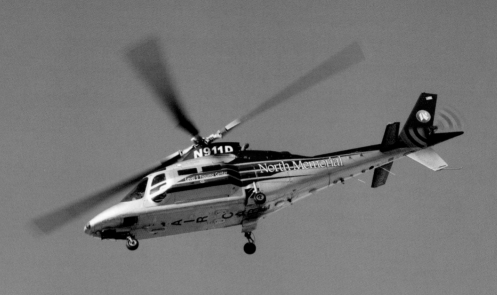

Sometimes patients have to be airlifted to hospitals for the proper medical care.

Together with another doctor, Styner created a system called Advanced Trauma Life Support. With this system, health-care workers quickly examine an injured patient. They provide basic care, such as bandaging wounds. Then they figure out what extra care is needed. If the hospital or clinic cannot provide the proper care, staff arrange for an ambulance or aircraft to take the patient to a better-equipped hospital. Clinics and hospitals in nearly ninety countries use this system. It has saved thousands of lives.

The Road to Failure

Gregor Mendel (*below left*) was a quiet man. Beginning in the 1850s, he taught science to high school students in Austria. He lived in a monastery, or religious community. He did experiments on pea plants in the monastery garden. Mendel studied how parent plants passed on traits to their offspring.

Mendel published a paper on his work in 1866, but few scientists paid attention. Some didn't understand his work with peas. Others said his theories were wrong. Mendel sent a copy of his paper to the famous British scientist Charles Darwin. Darwin didn't even open the package.

Mendel died in 1884. His work with genetics was forgotten. But in 1900, more than thirty years after he published his paper, other scientists finally paid attention. They realized that Mendel's ideas about genetics were right. His work is the basis for the modern study of genetics.

Chapter 4

SLIPS OF THE KNIFE

Fifty-two-year-old Willie King suffered from diabetes. In 1995, the disease damaged the blood vessels in his right leg. The leg became infected. To save King's life, doctors needed to amputate the leg.

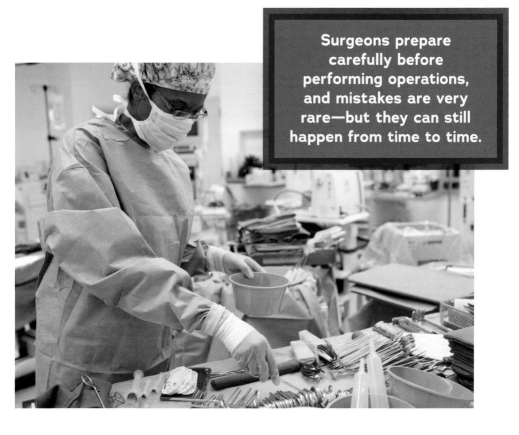

Surgeons prepare carefully before performing operations, and mistakes are very rare—but they can still happen from time to time.

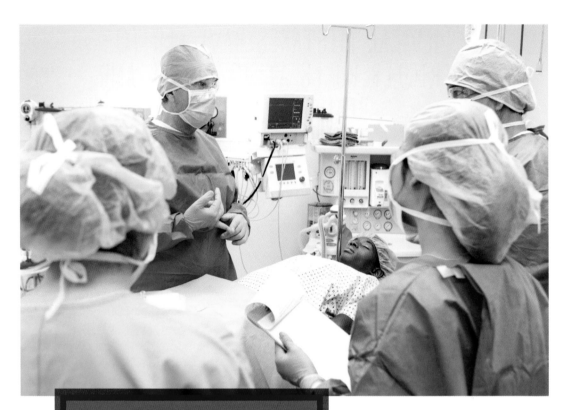

Mistakes in the operating room can make the difference between life and death.

King went to a hospital in Tampa, Florida, for the amputation. But on the chalkboard in the operating room, someone had written that his left leg was to be cut off. The hospital's computer system and the operating room schedule also listed the wrong leg. So the surgeon cut off the healthy leg.

MEDICAL MISTAKES HAVE LED TO STRICTER RULES AT HOSPITALS AND HEALTH CLINICS.

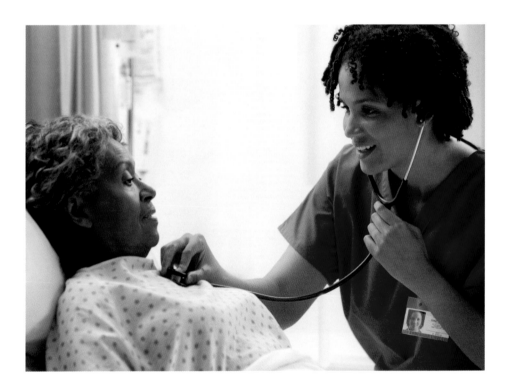

Because of this mistake, the hospital and the State of Florida wrote new procedures for operations. These procedures include computerized tracking systems and double-checking to make sure that doctors operate on the correct body parts.

Medical Souvenirs

In 2000, Donald Church underwent surgery at a medical center in Washington. During the operation, doctors removed a tumor from Church's stomach. But before the doctors closed his incision, they accidentally left a large surgical tool in his body.

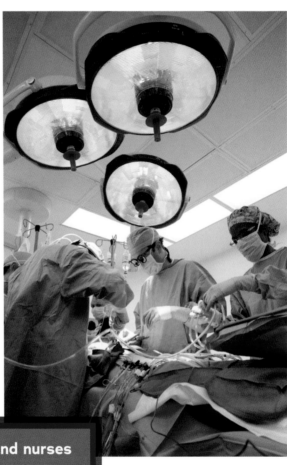

Doctors and nurses perform surgery.

Church experienced severe pain during recovery. With an X-ray, doctors discovered their mistake. They operated again to remove the tool.

An X-ray revealed a doctor's mistake: a surgical tool left inside the patient.

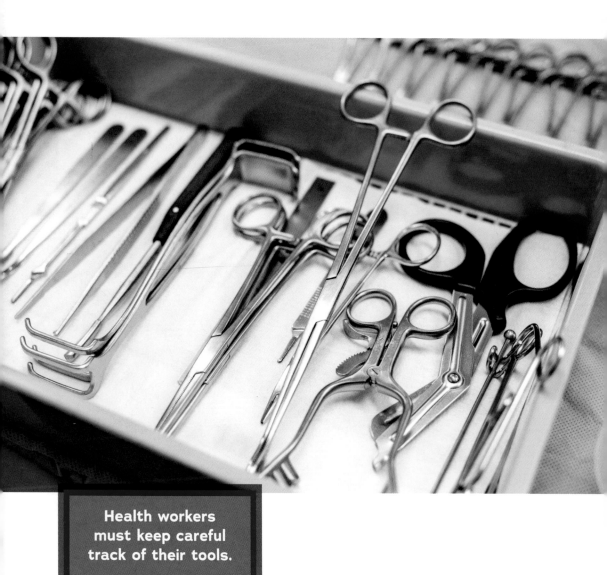

Health workers must keep careful track of their tools.

To prevent future mistakes, the medical center created new procedures. These include counting tools before and after surgery and taking X-rays of patients after surgery.

On the Cutting Edge

Doctors and scientists have worked hard to find new cures and relieve patient suffering. But they have also made mistakes. A Johns Hopkins University study said medical errors cause 9.5 percent of deaths in the United States.

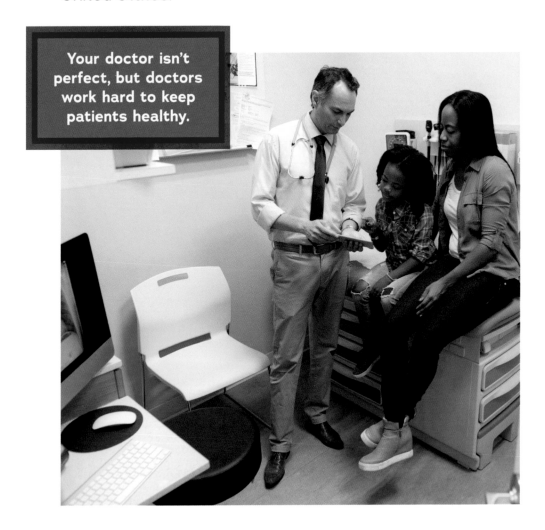

Your doctor isn't perfect, but doctors work hard to keep patients healthy.

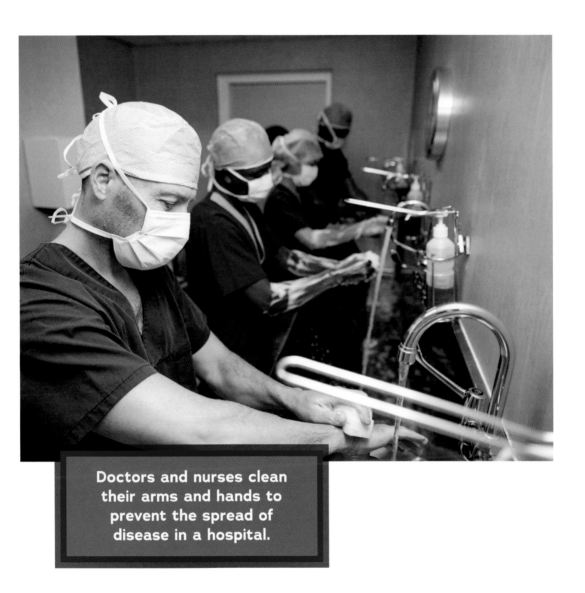

Doctors and nurses clean their arms and hands to prevent the spread of disease in a hospital.

But not all medical mistakes are bad. Without mistakes and accidents, we might not have X-rays. We might not have tiny, lifesaving pacemakers. We all make mistakes. The good news is that we can learn from them.

Glossary

amputation: the surgical removal of a body part, such as an arm or a leg

antibiotic: a substance that kills disease-causing bacteria

bacteria: tiny organisms found in air, water, and soil, and on the bodies of living things. Some bacteria cause diseases.

genetics: the study of how living things pass down traits to their offspring

implant: to insert something, such as a medical device, inside the body

incision: a cut in the body made by a surgeon

theory: an explanation or idea put forth for further investigation

transistor: a tiny device that controls a flow of electric current

vacuum tube: a glass or metal tube with all the air removed

virus: a tiny organism that can infect and sicken living things

X-ray: pictures of bones and internal organs, made using energy that can pass through skin and muscle

Learn More about Medicine Fails

Books

Farndon, John. *Strange Medicine: A History of Medical Remedies.* Minneapolis: Hungry Tomato, 2017. In earlier eras, doctors treated people with strange and slimy potions. Find out which ones worked and which ones didn't in this history of medical remedies.

Farndon, John. *Tiny Killers: When Bacteria and Viruses Attack.* Minneapolis: Hungry Tomato, 2017. This book explains how tiny germs can make us sick. It also tells how people learned to fight germs to keep themselves healthy.

Zuchora-Walske, Christine. *Your Head Shape Reveals Your Personality! Science's Biggest Mistakes about the Human Body.* Minneapolis: Lerner Publications, 2015. Long ago, doctors didn't understand how the human body worked. Read about some of their mistaken ideas.

Websites

BAM! Body and Mind
https://www.cdc.gov/bam/index.html
The US Centers for Disease Control and Prevention site offers games, quizzes, and tips about staying healthy.

Going to the Doctor
https://kidshealth.org/en/kids/going-to-dr.html
Even though doctors can make mistakes, kids still need to get regular checkups to stay healthy. Read about checkups, shots, and more.

How the Body Works
https://kidshealth.org/en/kids/center/htbw-main-page.html?WT.ac=k
-nav-htbw-main-page
Play games and learn more about your heart, brain, muscles, skin, and other body parts.

Index

Photo Acknowledgments

Image credits: Edward Savage, George Washington, Gift of Henry Prather Fletcher, National Gallery of Art, Washington DC, p. 4; Benjamin Henry Latrobe/Wikipedia, p. 5; Quirijn van Brekelenkam, The Bloodletting, Mauritshuis Museum CC 4.0, p. 6; Library of Congress LC-USZC4-10341, p. 7; CDC/NIAID, p. 8; Stock Montage/Getty Images, p. 9; monkeybusinessimages/Getty Images, p. 10; Photos.com/Getty Images, p. 11; Culture Club/Getty Images, p. 12; Wellcome Collection. CC by 4.0, pp. 13, 21; Radu Bercan/Shutterstock.com, p. 14; AP Photo/Bill Sikes, p. 15; Don Farrall/Digital Vision/Getty Images, p. 16; Bettmann/Getty Images, p. 17; sharply_done/Getty Images, p. 18; egdigital/Getty Images, p. 19; BanksPhotos/Getty Images, p. 20; ER Productions Limited/Getty Images, pp. 22, 25; Steve Debenport/Getty Images, p. 23; Jose Luis Pelaez Inc/Getty Images, p. 24; Peter Dazeley/Photographer's Choice/Getty Images, p. 26; JohnnyGreig/Getty Images, p. 27; Hero Images/Getty Images, p. 28; laflorGetty Images, p. 29.

Cover: BraunS/E+/Getty Images.